Praise for *Mother/Daughter Sex Advice*

What Everyone is Saying....
About Susie and Aretha Bright's
Mother/Daughter Sex Advice:

JEZEBEL.COM READERS:

I0436999

MEMO:
To: Jezebel Editors
From: Jezebel Readers
RE: Ms. Bright (and daughter Aretha)

It has come to our attention that you have started a series of posts wherein Ms. Bright (and daughter Aretha) answer readers' questions about assorted sexual topics and give overall advice regarding said topics.

These posts have proven to be insightful, informative, and entertaining.

We heartily recommend that this become a regular recurring feature on *Jezebel*; perhaps weekly like "Pot Psychology."

Thank you in advance for your consideration of this and we look forward to a positive response regarding this matter.

— AIDELMAIDEL

That was astonishing, and makes me want to go upstairs and promise my two sleeping little girls that I will be as good a mother as Ms. Bright clearly is. And I will totally be buying her book.

— QUEENJULIE

These two are stomach turning. There are some things that should not be shared between parent and child. — CHIC NOIR

Hey, *CHIC NOIR*: Honestly, I WISH my parents had been more upfront with me about sex—it would have made all the difference. So many parents pretend that they themselves don't have sex or never did before marriage, or just don't address the topic at all, which in turn makes their children not want to communicate about sex—or makes them feel the need to be secretive or feel that sex is shameful. I don't think Susie and Aretha's relationship is for EVERYONE, but it's certainly healthy and definitely awesome that they feel comfortable being so open. —ANTISOCIALSOCIALITY

CHIC NOIR: Yep—"stomach turning" is the first word that popped into my head when I read their easygoing, joking comments and reasonable, helpful responses. —APRILLAYNE

This was so inspiring (and made me get all teary). I hope I can do half this well when the time comes. —RESPLENDENT.BITCH

Although it sometimes makes me uneasy when I think about the fact that they are mother and daughter, it also inspires a bit of jealousy - I wish I could discuss some of these issues with my own mother with even a fraction of the honesty and frankness they share.

—HELEN SKOR

Love this. I hope my son grows up to find me safe and trustworthy enough that he could come to me for any kind of help. Susie and Aretha have a good thing going. —RITUALTHEORY

Right ON Susie and Aretha! Sex-education starts at home. :) —XAN'TSTOPWON'TSTOP

THIS RULES! —ZAP ROWSDO

I'm not gonna lie. I'm jealous of you, Aretha. —BESARCASTIC

MOTHER/DAUGHTER SEX ADVICE

MOTHER/DAUGHTER

SEX ADVICE

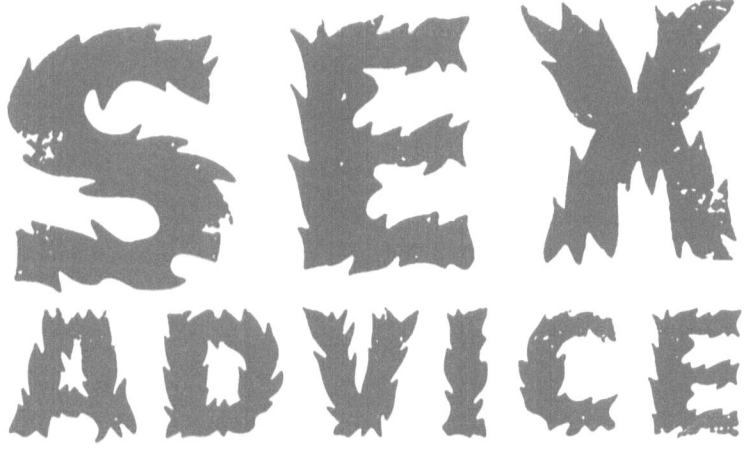

SUSIE & ARETHA

BRIGHT

Bright Stuff

CONTENTS

WHAT'S IT LIKE...
TO WRITE A MOTHER/DAUGHTER
SEX ADVICE COLUMN?

In 2009, Jezebel.com, a popular women's blog, asked Susie Bright (52) and Aretha Bright (19) to write a guest sex advice column responding to their readers' questions. This is what happened...

INTRODUCTION FROM THE DAUGHTER

My mom likes to work in bed. It's not uncommon to see her laying on her bed, backed by millions of pillows, typing away on her computer. I usually barge right in and flop down. (Sometimes she likes the company, other times she lets me know I'm not welcome).

On one such occasion, she asked me if I wanted to help her with a work project—she said it would be really fun. As soon as I found out that it was "answering people's sex problems," I jumped on board. I love giving advice!

Usually I don't have enough people to give advice to, but this time I got to sift through a bunch of *Dear Susie...* emails with my mom, and decide which ones we would feature in the column. My instinct was to answer all of them.

My mom and I have read aloud advice columns together for a long time, everything from *Dear Abby, Dear Prudence...* to eventually, *Dear Dan Savage*. I loved disagreeing with the more conservative advice columnists, and ate up the intimate details and wilder material in Dan's column or other "adult" magazines. The people who wrote us at *Jezebel* tended to disclose more, which was helpful— the more details, the better.

The reaction that we got from *Jezebel* readers was super-mixed. Some applauded us for our wonderful mother-daughter relationship, and commented on how funny and witty we were. (Ego stroke!) Others found the idea of mother/daughter sex conversation disgusting or uncomfortable. I felt immune to that particular criticism because I had grown up my whole life with sex being an ordinary topic in my household and extended family.

There was one strand of *Jezebel* comments that insisted that my mom shouldn't be proud of me—because what kind of mother would want a daughter who was so sexually experienced by age 18, that she could give advice?

Well, I never talked about the amount of personal sexual experience I had had. Insight and knowledge from growing up in an environment where relationships, sex, and politics were discussed in both informal and intellectual ways. I don't think that's typical. However, I think young people—teenagers in particular—have A LOT more wisdom and savvy intuition than people give us credit for. I'd encourage anyone to talk about sex and not feel inhibited, regardless of their relationship experience.

Once our advice column debuted, the letters started pouring in. At the same time, I moved from my home to college, a couple hours away, so Susie and I couldn't always replicate the "writing room" on her bed. Sometimes we did columns over the phone. Afterward, one of us would be in charge of writing up the notes, and edit it for our column format.

Although our columns give a realistic feel of what was said, there was actually a lot more talking over each other, groaning, laughing, and random conversations in between.

We answered three people a week, but that never seemed like enough for me. I wanted to do more like *twenty*. Everyone who wrote us sounded so sympathetic and nice; I felt a special connection with them. Although sometimes our reactions were flip or sassy (some of which are embarrassing for me to look at now) I really did care about everyone who asked for our help.

I was obsessed with checking our column once it was published. I read the comments as they came in, sometimes by the minute. *Jezebel* readers are ready to be ruthless (I say that as a *Jezebel* reader myself)—and they can pile onto any little thing. A few commenters would criticize a small point that Susie or I said, and I would be devastated. I took it personally, and even though I knew it would "make things worse" if I rebutted every nit-pick, I was dying to defend myself, to explain the misunderstanding. "No, really, I didn't say that a girl should RAPE her boyfriend!"

Yes, I did cry on a few occasions.

Fortunately, most readers loved our column, and had kind or interesting things to add to the discussion. But there was one commenter who reee-ally had it in for us. "Anonymous," of course; I never knew who it was. Even though s/he attacked us repeatedly on every issue, and said from the start that we did not belong on *Jezebel*, this mystery critic read every single word we wrote. Each week, I waited for his or her criticism, looked for their avatar icon. I waited to see if there would be a crusade against us this week, or just snide comments. Since our column ended, I've looked for "Our Troll" else-where on *Jezebel*, but s/he has disappeared. Hmmm...

I also liked to watch the traffic on our weekly post, and compare it to other articles that debuted the same day. I'd get grumpy if some-thing big happened in the news on "our Wednesday." I panicked if our column wasn't at the top of the news feed for more than six hours. So neurotic. It's kind of cute to think about now.

Looking back at our columns, I'm proud of the work we did. Just like having sex for the first time, being a sex-advice columnist for the first time is a unique experience you can't replicate. I'd like to thank everyone who supported us, the fans, *Jezebel*, and editor Anna Holmes for giving us the platform. Most of all, I'd like to thank my mom for giving me the opportunity, and for always giving me the best advice about anything.

ARETHA BRIGHT
February, 2012

THE FIRST PANCAKE

DEAR ARETHA AND SUSIE,

I am about to have sex with someone and it is his first time. He is very nervous and loses his erection every time we begin to put a condom on. Help!
—**Kitty**

ARETHA: A girl after my own heart! First, on the condoms—make sure they're the easiest, roomiest, most user-friendly you can buy. Like, *"Twisted Pleasure Trojan,"* or *"Her Pleasure."*

SUSIE: I swear by the "P"-shaped condoms, like the *"Pleasure Plus,"* or the *"Lifestyle Dual Pleasure."*

ARETHA: Trojan is everywhere. The point is, no *"Kimono Micro Thin"* or that cheap crap they hand out at the college nurse's office.

Tell him, however you want to say it: "You're going to masturbate with condoms." You get him to "Jack and Edge," that's the homework.

SUSIE: Did you make that up? "Jack and Edge"? I mean, I know what you mean, instantly, but I have never heard that before.

ARETHA: Yeah, that's what I decided to call it.

SUSIE: Everyone else calls it "stop and start" or something clinical, but this is much better.

ARETHA: Once he gets the good ones, he needs to learn he can come with them on, so he can put "condom and coming" together. That won't take long.

The next part is: whatever gets him off, before intercourse, you have to do that a lot. If you haven't already, say all the reassuring stuff like: "It's going to be fun, good for me, fun for you, etc."

The first pancake, it's like that. You're going to make a lot more and the second one will be better. It doesn't matter if he comes right away—it's like, "Don't worry, we'll do it again and again."

Now, depending on his type, you might have to be the girl who gets him hard, puts the condom on him right then, sits down on him, and starts moving. That's if he needs to be pounced on. But if he has to make the first move, then you have to start out really relaxed, no rush—pretend like you could be doing anything. You have an open invitation to have sex, but no focus on, "We're going to have sex in the next five minutes." One time, in this situation, I even took a "little nap." Once my attention was off of the guy, he recharged and went for it.

But then there's you, how you get ready. You better masturbate that day beforehand, because the deflowering is probably going to be about him, not you. Take care of yourself so you can relax. This could take more than one date. It's real important not to get focused on one night. If it's a holiday, or one of those "special occasions," make it easy and romantic, nothing too difficult to put together, 'cause that's too much pressure. Three candles, some good food, whatever, but just keep trying.

SUSIE: Okay, but what if you do all that, and his erection fails when he actually is about to enter you?

ARETHA: Take the condom off immediately. Start jacking or touching him; say, "I'm so glad you have a lot of condoms, we're going to go through a lot!"

"MY BOYFRIEND SAYS HE'S MESSY WHEN IT COMES TO ORAL SEX"

DEAR ARETHA AND SUSIE,

My BF really wants to come in my mouth. I'm nervous about this because he says he's very messy. What should I be expecting? Is it a shooting feeling? A squirt-from-a-water-bottle feeling? I want to give him this experience but I'm afraid I'm going to end up choking or something equally disastrous. I've already gagged a couple of times after being a bit too adventurous. I do want to try it but I'm so scared!

—Claire

ARETHA: Are you SURE you want to try it? [Laughing] I think your boyfriend could be reassuring you a bit more. Does he know this is how you feel about it?

SUSIE: "Very messy?" Compared to what? I think guys exaggerate, 'cause most of them haven't seen a lot of other guys come!

ARETHA: Okay, FIRST—he could come earlier in the day, before you see each other, so that there isn't as much to deal with. The force isn't bad.

SUSIE: We're not talking about a fire hose; this is like a couple tablespoons at most.

ARETHA: Just a couple splats. Now, the taste is probably not going to thrill you—that's the thing that might make you gag, not the force of the ejaculation. Get ready to not like it. (Although there are exceptions!)

SUSIE: It isn't ice cream. Here's the exciting part: If you like the feeling of having someone lose control with you, you're going to love this! You won't know until you try it. It can be a real rush if you understand how much power you have. Have at least one hand on his cock so you can control it. If you start to choke, just pull back.

ARETHA: Yeah—and just because he comes in your mouth, you don't have to swallow... although that will get it out of your mouth the fastest. Not too big a deal and if gets messy or whatever you can laugh about it. Have fun!

HIGH SCHOOL PORN STAR

A girl I went to high school with is a porn star now. She was always stunningly beautiful and nice to everyone then—and she's still both of those things. She loves what she does and is successful. I'm happy for her.

It makes me feel bad, though, when I come across her videos and see captions calling her derogatory names. What steps are being taken so that more movies where girls are having fun and are in charge are made? What other steps are being taken so that porn stars can be viewed as human beings? Do you think it is possible for porn to evolve in this direction?   **—Sherryl**

ARETHA: Uh, I think porn *already* has changed a lot. For a long time! I mean, there are women directors and feminist porn…if she were working with different people, they wouldn't be treating her bad. (Check out Cathy Winks' *Guide to Adult Videos*).

SUSIE: Have you talked to her about it? Why do *you* keep watching? I don't know what the deal is with you two. If you're close, you would talk about this stuff. If you're not, you're a voyeur. But here's something to remember: If she were in Hollywood movies or primetime TV, you might also be shocked and disgusted at all the sexist degrading things that she was being put through. It's not any different just because you're naked and screwing.

ARETHA: That's a good point. I mean, take "Kim Bauer!"

SUSIE: You mean, the annoying daughter from the 24 show? Yeah, it doesn't get worse than that

"CAN A WOMAN COME FROM INTERCOURSE ALONE?"

DEAR SUSIE & ARETHA,

Where do you get off, saying that a woman can't come from intercourse alone? I come from straight fucking without any problem, always have. Just because *you* have a problem doesn't mean everyone else does. My vagina has orgasms, not my clitoris. —*Carla*

SUSIE: I think we have a "word" problem. When I say that penis-vagina intercourse can't make a woman orgasm, I mean that the sensation of a phallus sliding against vaginal walls is not sufficient. If our vaginal walls were sensitive enough to spark orgasm, we would all suffer horrible deaths from sheer pain during childbirth. It's our birth canal!

When I insist, "There's got to be some clitoral stimulation, or there's no female orgasm," I'm talking about a very *big* understanding of the clit. It is a lot bigger than most people think. And you can't see most of it from the outside! There's certainly more than one way to make it happy.

Let's think about men's anatomy—everyone knows what a man's cock and balls look like. If you told a man that his "penis" was nothing more than the head of his cock—his "glans"—he would laugh in your face. If he pitied you, he might tell you that there was an important aspect to the penis called the shaft, also the frenulum, and perhaps a foreskin. His scrotum and balls are part of the essential package as well.

Women's anatomy education, on the other hand, has been a giant exercise in vacancy.

Until recent times, we've been schooled that the clitoris—the female analog to the penis—is nothing more than the small glans one can see on the outside of the vulva. Start laughing now! Women

6

have a big, big, clitoral body—but it's nearly all on the inside, instead of the outdoor plumbing that's viewed so easily on men.

The reason you hear so much about the "G-spot," and controversies over whether women are excited by internal anal or vaginal pressure, is because those areas are all means to massage, and stimulate, the *internal* clitoral body. The G-spot isn't some extra accessory; it's just one of many inches on the clitoral map. Remember: the whole clit, and nothing but.

Of course, the female clitoral glans is the super-sensitive part, just like a man's. But in the same way that men like to have their entire penises taken into account when they're aroused, women are favored by attention to their entire clitorises.

When I present this information in public, I am hampered by my lack of rendering skills. Now, finally, I have the genius of Betty "Quick Draw" Dodson to show you what's it's all about. The next time someone asks you, "Where's the clitoris? What does it look like? How do you know where to find it?" you simply come over here, and press play.

"I'M A VIRGIN—AND IT MEANS SOMETHING TO ME"

DEAR ARETHA AND SUSIE,

I'm 18, almost 19. I'm a virgin, but have been hooking up with a friend of mine named Andy for a few months. It recently went as far as mutual hand jobs and phalanges—penetration. He says he absolutely does not want a relationship. I know that our "arrangement" is not exclusive.

I would be very comfortable losing my virginity to him, but I'm stuck on the fact that I WOULD want a relationship.

He's been with five or six girls already. I'm afraid my virginity won't mean anything to him. I don't want it to mean *Everything*, but I need it to mean *Something* to the other person, because it would certainly mean *Something* to me.

The first time we hooked up, he told me, "If anything ever happens between us—and you need it to mean something, I can do that for you."

Do you think I should go ahead and lose my virginity to my friend—and get on with my life? Or should I wait until I find someone I'm comfortable around who actually wants a relationship?

—*Marguerite*

ARETHA: He says he can "do" this for you? That doesn't sound too generous. I'm not getting a good impression.

I've gone through this before—you're in a touchy situation, analyzing it all alone, and remembering "single sentences." You end up misleading yourself. It doesn't matter what he said when you first hooked up—it's different now.

SUSIE: I need a break from the romantic angst. Does he make you horny, as opposed to "comfortable?" When you make out with him, are you dying to do more? I can't emphasize how much that will make a difference in terms of your first time with him.

If you have great sex, you'll always be glad of that experience, even if the two of you don't ride off into the sunset. But if you have mediocre sex with Mr. Aloof, you will either get more hung-up on the unrequited romance, or you will tire of him.

BTW, Andy doesn't know what he'll feel like after he makes love with you—all this "planning" is rubbish. It's not that much under anyone's control.

ARETHA: I don't care what he "says." It will mean something to him; it always does.

SUSIE: Virginity is wildly overrated.

ARETHA: I agree with you about the virginity hype from a feminist p.o.v.—but virginity meant something to me—and it still seems important for most people. It's already SOMETHING for her; you can't argue that away.

SUSIE: But what is this "something"? It's obviously not about her hymen OR the true meaning of love OR the definitive erotic moment.

I'd love her to read Greta Christina's *"Are We Having Sex Now or Not?"*—Mandatory reading for "virgins." Ex-virgins, too.

Marguerite, follow your gut. If you know you're going to be heartbroken, forget it. Get those "fingers" out of your life.

"I'VE BEEN DATING
A TRANSMAN..."

DEAR ARETHA AND SUSIE,

I've been dating a transman for a while now, who lives as a male, but has not yet undergone any hormone or surgical transition. In the beginning, he loved sex between us and made it clear he identified as a straight man, exclusively.

Then, out of nowhere on our last vacation, he got drunk and kissed another GUY at the bar, which he blamed on booze.

Last night, drunk again, he said he thinks he might be into guys, but wants to be with me.

So, do I call it a day, not being a "guy" and all? I'm pretty old-fashioned and if he was a bio—dude, I'd say *sayonara* (and probably throw a "Hooray, You're Gay" party to be supportive).

Or, should I wait for him to bring this up when he's sober since he keeps blowing off the drunken gay-ness the next day when I ask about it?

—Allyson

ARETHA: You said he was loving the sex with you. Do you mean that after he kissed a guy, it all changed—or did your sex life go bad before that?

SUSIE: People get drunk and kiss other drunks all the time. But did it mean more to you at this stage, because your sex life was in the toilet?

It's only natural that things are going to get sloppy every once in a while, especially if your lover hasn't hashed everything out yet with his sexual feelings. Of course, he doesn't want to get "divorced" from you! You sound like his best friend. Did you witness the kissing or did he tell you about it? That's an important difference.

ARETHA: If he'd kissed another women, would you have a problem with that? Is this a jealousy thing or are you starting to feel like he's not into women anymore, period? I agree with Susie, it's too early in the game for either of you to decide whether he's "gay" or not. To the point, if the sex is sucking, who cares if he's gay, bi, or just naughty? Maybe it's time to leave.

"WILL I EVER GET USED TO ANAL SEX?"

DEAR ARETHA AND SUSIE,

I just started having anal sex with my boyfriend. We did it once. He is gentle and slow-going at it, because he doesn't want to hurt me.

Although it was a bit uncomfortable, I enjoyed the sensation of it. But I didn't come. If we have anal sex as little as once every couple months, will I get used to it?—and maybe come from it someday?

—*Jasmine*

ARETHA: Well, if you want to come from *anything* new, you're going to have to try it more than once every couple months. The first time, in part, could have been uncomfortable because it was unfamiliar.

SUSIE: I've glad he's gentle and slow…that means you can talk to him while it's happening. I like this guy already. He obviously has control of his erection, which makes a big difference! He'd love it if you talked to him. I know this is the sex educator mantra, but anal sex is about lubrication and communication—each one of those ideas is going to make a lot more sense the more you try it.

Gentle pressure from the anus or rectum can stimulate the "underbelly" of your clitoris; its internal body. But the glans of your clit is still the most sensitive part.

ARETHA: Yeah, you're not likely to orgasm from backdoor alone.

HUSBAND WANTS TO PUSH WIFE OFF ORGASM CLIFF

DEAR ARETHA AND SUSIE,

My wife gets "to the peak "during intercourse and will not go over the edge. She'll beg me to keep going, "don't stop, keep going"—but even during those times when I can, in fact, keep it going—she never orgasms from intercourse alone. But I swear, she is on the edge of that orgasm. How do I get her over that edge? *—Peter*

SUSIE: Of course she doesn't come "from intercourse alone." No woman does. I'd love to strike that phrase from the English language.

ARETHA: Put your hand down there! Or one of those vibrators that slip on your finger like a ring!

SUSIE: It's the same dilemma as if she licked your balls and the bottom of your shaft for hours… you'd be screaming for relief, too. You'd need some serious attention to the head of your cock, just like virtually every other man in the universe.

You know, the answer is a lot closer than you think. How does your wife masturbate? How does she make herself come? Does she use something like a dildo—like inside her? How does she get over the top? She knows. Ask her sometime when you're nowhere near the sexual tension bubble.

"I HAVE A TENDENCY TO THROW UP EVERY TIME MY BOYFRIEND COMES IN MY MOUTH"

DEAR ARETHA AND SUSIE,

I have a tendency to throw up every single time my boyfriend comes in my mouth. I'm not sure if it's my gag reflex or the taste that causes it. Is there anything I can do to try and stop myself from throwing up?

—*Wretched*

ARETHA: Stop having your boyfriend come in your mouth, Number #1. Why does this keep going on?

SUSIE: Are you gagging, or vomiting up food? Good grief; it's non-consensual S/M. Do you mind this sensation, or you're just concerned about appearances? Or are you bragging? A tiny bit of gagging can be "cute" if you have total control over it. If you want to do the fantasy where you act like, "Oh, Mr. Big, I couldn't possibly...!"

ARETHA: (Stare)

SUSIE: Aretha, stop looking at me like I'm crazy; this is a fantasy some people play out. But if the girl means she's really retching, it isn't funny.

ARETHA: Wretched, am I detecting that your boyfriend really likes it, and you're just trying to cope with it? Doesn't he *mind* that you throw up? How is that *not* turning him off? Is he *choking* on your vagina? Are you getting some action too?

SUSIE: We can't tell, we don't know. It's kinda mysterious the way she puts it.

ARETHA: If you had the opportunity to never have to give a blow job again, unless you were wild about it, how would that make you feel? Pretend your boyfriend had no particular interest in it, and it was only your whim.

SUSIE: Some women want to be able to please their lovers orally, just to have it in their "toolbox" of techniques, but they really can't stand deep throat, or taking come in their mouths.

If that's the case, you want to control his penis with one or both of your hands so you can pull it out, exactly how and when you please. The last three seconds, when he's coming, he's not going to be paying a lot of detailed attention to whether he's in your mouth or in your hands. If it's the taste that's the only problem, you need to anticipate his ejaculation, and pull it out. Maybe you'd like to get fancy with your licking techniques.

ARETHA: TMI, Mom!

SUSIE: ...Yes, thank you Aretha, but I'm not being personal, just hear me out. Many men like to be "licked" just as much or more as being "sucked," and if more women know that, they wouldn't go through all the angst.

ARETHA: You never hear a guy asking you to "lick" him!

SUSIE: Now I'm going to stare at you. This isn't a Hollywood movie. It's real life. Some guys have never tried it. A lot of them don't ask for anything—they're stoic. The point is, try it. What have you got to lose?

ARETHA: There is the chance that this guy's semen is unusually bad-tasting. What does he eat? It's got to *stop*!

SUSIE: Pineapple: good; asparagus: bad. Or you could deep throat for real and miss out on the taste altogether.

ARETHA: I can't take this anymore.

"GROSS FOR SOME PEOPLE..."

DEAR ARETHA AND SUSIE,

Okay, this may be gross for some people, but I have to ask. My boy-friend has expressed an interest in being peed and shat on. I'm curious to try this out but I have no idea how to do it at all. I know how to go to the bathroom, obviously, but I mean in a sexy, clean, fun way for both of us—and also with minimal clean-up if possible. Any suggestions? Also, I am wondering where this interest comes from for people? Is it Freudian or is it as simple as just wanting to try new and different things sexually?

—**Rose**

ARETHA: Mom, I DON'T KNOW! What happens to the *shit*? Do you do it in shower? What is the right setting?

SUSIE: The bathroom is the right place; you've got that right. The pee is not really that big of a deal, it's sterile, you've probably peed in the shower before and never even thought about it.

ARETHA: My default answer to *all* sex questions is light some candles and it'll be a lot sexier. Bubble bath, maybe!

SUSIE: Dealing with scat makes things a lot more medical, you have to put on your nurse hat and really plan things, to avoid infection. I would treat these two things apart from each other. The pee could be an easy experiment without a lot of risk—and then you could see how you felt about his fantasy, and the whole psychological side of it, with him. Here's a couple of highly informative books: *Anal Pleasure and Health*, and *Intimate Invasion: The Erotic Ins & Outs of Enema Play*.

You could ask where his fantasy comes from…you could ask that about anything. Why do people want to do it in the missionary position, aside from peer pressure? Why do people make porn out of anything and every subject? Fetish usually comes from memories, like every part of our unconscious. The hidden issue behind your question is that he wants you to dominate him and revel in humiliation…you have to find out how you jibe with that, regardless of the bodily fluids.

"I'M 27 YEARS OLD AND I'VE NEVER HAD AN ORGASM"

DEAR ARETHA AND SUSIE,

I'm 27 and have never had an orgasm. Not alone, not with someone else. My girlfriends' advice to "get to know my body" and "relax" hasn't evolved since I was 19. I am relaxed and I DO masturbate—plenty!

Most of the men I've slept with say, "Wow, even without an orgasm you sure are enjoying it!" Things like that. One of my longterm partners thinks I enjoy sex more than most women he's been with; I just don't orgasm. Once, I had a "mini-orgasm," as I like to refer to it. My legs went a little numb and I didn't want to move—the pleasure was really great—and then my whole body shivered and I had to lay down for lack of energy.

That's what I've gathered an orgasm is like, except that on the pleasure scale, this was a 5 out of the 10 that I normally experience with good penetration sex. Any advice? Is this more common than I think? Was my mini-orgasm really an orgasm? —*Almost There*

ARETHA: We all want to know: What does a "10" in penetration sex feel like?

SUSIE: Yes, that's the focus for me. What makes the fucking part feels so good? Details, please! What were you doing when the little sun burst out? If you combined whatever that was, with the fucking you like, it would the perfect combo.

ARETHA: Remember how Ducky Doolittle was telling us how she gave herself mini- orgasms when she was a little girl by flexing her Kegel muscles, which led to much stronger orgasms over time?

SUSIE: Yes, the minis are definitely foreplay for what's to come.

ARETHA: We don't know how your masturbating, but if you like penetration, get a nice dildo and a *Magic Wand*, turn it on full blast and see if anything happens. The penetration you like, plus the vibrator, might push you over the edge. You don't want to get "relaxed"—you want to get excited. Important difference. Sometimes people feel inhibited and that gets translated as "not relaxing," but "tense," as in "really horny" is very, very good.

SUSIE: About your age... there's no age that's "normal" for figuring out your sexual zenith. There's women twice your age who haven't had half the pleasure you've discovered so far. Don't let those thoughts occupy your mind.

ARETHA: It's hard when you're trying to make your body cooperate on a schedule. In Jennifer Lehr's book, *Ill—Equipped for a Life of Sex*, the husband and wife had to schedule sex dates because their love life was so awful—it was so inorganic and forced. She described so well how trying too hard is a disaster. I don't want you to feel like, "Back to homework!" Get horny, follow your hottest fantasies, your craziest suggestions to your lover—the sole pursuit of pleasure—rather than, "I'll work on my Orgasm Project Today." Don't take the fun out of it just because you're in a hurry for it to happen. I hope an "11" takes you by surprise very, very soon!

BIG GAMETES JUST WANNA HAVE FUN

Aretha took her first Junior semester at San Francisco State University, where she TA'ed a 750-students-enrolled sex education class. The class uses a lot of tech that frequently breaks... and one of the remote mikes shorted out during the extra-credit question period of a recent mid-term exam.

The question was:
   "Species-wide, what makes females "female" and males "male"? Is it:

A. that males have testes and females don't?

B. that females lactate and males don't?

C. that males possess the "xy" chromosome and females the "xx"?

D. that males have small gametes and females have large gametes?

E. that females prefer monogamy more than males?

   Aretha would like you to know that to her amazement, eight students picked (e), which is incorrect, both biologically and politically.

   But the question *is* tricky if you haven't studied species-wide sexuality. Now, the true answers can now be revealed!
   Is it...
A. that males have testes and females don't?

   Wrong. For example, Spotted Hyena females all have "penises" and a scrotum.

B. that females lactate and males don't?

Wrong. Male Indonesian Fruit Bats lactate milk.

C. that males possess the "xy" chromosome and females the "xx"?

Wrong. Chickens don't even have XY chromosomes.

D. that males have small gametes and females have large gametes?

Correct! Congratulations, Smarty Pants!

A whopping 30% of quiz-takers at *Jezebel* picked the correct answer. And they're a smart crowd—it's really a problem that Americans don't get more science education these days.

The most popular answer, albeit wrong, was that old "chromosome" canard. That was followed by a couple dozen entries that fell for the testes gambit, and only one curiosity seeker who chose "lactation"—guess everyone knew about the fruit bats.

One last shocker: the correct answers came from a disproportionately high number of Canadian and UK Jezebel readers. Read it and weep, Yankees!

THE BOY WHO DIDN'T LIKE DOGGIE

DEAR ARETHA AND SUSIE,
I like being fucked from behind, but my boyfriend refuses to even try it. He says it's gross, that it's for dogs, not people. What can I do to persuade him that it's fun, and not an insult?   **—Alessandra**

ARETHA: He's the problem. What's the matter with him?? Ummm... maybe he should watch A *Snoop Dogg* video.

SUSIE: Jesus, how do you even know about that title? No, don't tell me—I don't want to know.

ARETHA: Well, I didn't want to hear you answer that other masturbation question!

SUSIE: Okay, let's start over. We agreed we could both say "TMI" whenever we wanted to. How do we get this boyfriend to not be so uptight?

ARETHA: I'd probably get a little evil.

SUSIE: You mean, trick him?

ARETHA: Yeah, you lay down and say you want a back massage, "Just a back massage." So then he has to straddle you, so he can do it right. That gets him used to being relaxed on top of you. Look back at him, give him lots of eye contact and encouragement. Ask him to bite your neck. He's just got to get comfortable being back there. You'll feel his comfort level coming up, and then you just make it happen. If all fails, just sit on him backwards, and slip it in.

SUSIE: You make it sound so simple. But you're probably right. I have to guess this is a young man. I don't think this phase of his is going to last very long. He probably thinks all kinds of things are gross, like green vegetables, but pretty soon he's going to grow up.

DUMPED AFTER 4 YEARS...
AND STILL A VIRGIN

DEAR ARETHA & SUSIE,

Recently, I was ditched in a four-year sexually-awesome relationship. During our time together, the ex and I had mad hot, kinky, crazy times.

The problem? Now that I've been dumped, I've been freaking out about the fact that I'm still a "virgin." I don't know how much I buy this virginity nonsense, having enjoyed my sex plenty of times with partners and no penetration involved. But now that I'm alone and thinking I'm never going to meet another partner like him, I'm wondering what's going to happen to me.

Oh, and the main reason for my "virginity" and non-penetration so far? Yes, I'm scared (due to reoccurring rape dreams since I was eleven) and it hurts. Like, a lot. I had a moment where I was so frustrated, that I tried to just DIY it with my cute little vibrator, and just... nothing. Even post-shower, tons of porn, and a good hour of stimulation.

Is it okay to be a "virgin" forever? Or do I need to just lose it, even if it hurts like crazy- so I can catch up and not be freaking myself out? *Craigslist* has not been the most helpful during this time.

—Like a Virgin

SUSIE: You're right, you're not a virgin if what that means is sexual experience. There are lots of women who don't have "intact hymens" who have not had nearly as much sex, or as pleasurable sex, as you have!

While you were with your old boyfriend, your sex pattern kept your mind off the real issue, which is, "Why does vaginal penetration hurt so much?" But now it's front and center. You have to get to the bottom of this, for your own sake.

ARETHA: It sounds like you may have an particularly-thick hymen; not everybody's is the same. Tearing your hymen might hurt some, but what you're talking about seems a little extreme. No success after an hour of stimulation? You did all the right things, but something else is going on.

SUSIE: Forget Craigslist, it's time to see a gynecologist! I don't always parrot, "See a doctor, see a therapist"—but in this case, you need some experienced, sympathetic, pros. Have you had an OBGYN exam before?

The gyno would be able to see what's up with your hymen. You may also be dealing with vaginismus; it's not an unusual condition. It's when your PC muscle clenches, involuntarily, so tight, that any kind of penetration is impossible. It can get to be a vicious circle, because if you fear the pain, and then try to push past it- only to experience worse—you're going feel even more apprehension.

There's treatment that is very effective, called "systematic dilation" - a more gentle, gradual version of the masturbation you tried. But you need to get a visual of what's up with your hymen.

ARETHA: Hold on—you've been having frightening rape dreams since you were eleven? It's hard to point the finger in these cases, but that is a pretty haunting memory. Do you have them nowadays—have you talked to anyone about them?

I know money is an issue for everyone now, but I definitely think you should see a therapist—your rape dreams might reveal more about why you feel so inhibited about penetration. You wrote us, so I know you don't want to be alone with this - that's the right instinct!

THE COMMON HOUSEHOLD
SEX TOY

DEAR ARETHA & SUSIE,

This is probably a really stupid question, but here goes...

I've never bought a sex toy before, and was happy using my hands—they were doing a great job on their own. But a few nights ago, I wanted something to add to it all—and for some reason, dug out my hairbrush and used it. It is perfect for hitting my g-spot (the handle is curved and ribbed; ingenious, no?) I've hardly been able to stop since I discovered it.

However, now I'm worried. No one else uses my hairbrush, but what if they wanted to? Would I have to stop them and (not) tell them why? Can I catch anything from brushing my head with the same brush?

I'm kind of broke, which is why I haven't bought something specifically for the task yet. I feel like I should probably buy two brushes. Having said that, I work hard and have little time to myself—so I don't know that I can be bothered to go buy another hair brush.

Should I just keep the one brush super clean and have it as my little secret?

—*Kate*

SUSIE: The only thing that's even a tiny bit "stupid" about your question is that you NEGLECTED to tell us the make and model of your hair brush!

It's refreshing to hear someone find their own "sex toys" around the house or in the garden, instead of spending ridiculous amounts of money. When I first sold vibrators in 1980, we sold the basic battery model for... hold your breath... ninety-nine cents. I feel like Grandma Horse-and-Buggy.

You're in a long line of women who have found that their comb, toothbrush, shampoo bottle, and the edge of the washing machine can offer a gal a real good time.

ARETHA: I didn't even realize until recently that it was so expensive to buy sex toys, because you always had these "samples" coming to the house in the mail and you'd stash them in your office. It was like a never-ending supply. Remember when I got my hands on one of your sample dildos, and cut it in half with a scissors?

SUSIE: What?

ARETHA: It was the really pretty blue and white swirly one. I had to see what it looked like inside.

SUSIE: Wait—how long ago was this? You were like eight or nine, right? Oh yeah, I remember—it was one of those silicon numbers that looked like a candy cane.

ARETHA: I used it to play with my Barbies. It was the sex "totem pole" that all my Barbies succumbed to. The Barbies were my special hero agents that would fight the evil totem pole. It was about their height, so it was just right for a character in Barbie World.

SUSIE: Why was it evil?

ARETHA: Umm, I think I knew I wasn't supposed to have it, so I made it a "bad character..."

SUSIE: How did you get busted? I can only remember the part where I held up the shreds in disbelief.

ARETHA: I hadn't cleaned up my room or something, and you or Dad came in to nag me to put the Barbie Village away—and then you saw this cut-up dildo on the floor: "Oh my god!"

SUSIE: Kate, we thank you for bringing back these treasured memories!

Now back to the nitty-gritty of your question: The only criteria to use when you judge an impromptu sex toy, is to make sure it's perfectly smooth, with no sharp edges or seams. Vaginally, it can be any shape you like, since your vag is a cul-de-sac. But if you ever want to use something for anal penetration, you need to make sure it has a flange (flared base). In that case, you hairbrush is fine for that, too.

If you want to use your "found dildo" more than once, just make sure it's washable, non-porous. If it would survive a spin in the dishwasher, it's a good candidate. Your hairbrush is probably hard plastic, which is ideal.

Where's all your apprehension coming from, after your fun? Honestly, how many times do people stomp into your bedroom and demand to use your hairbrush?

ARETHA: Like never. Listen, Kate: If you don't want people to use your brush, JUST SAY NO. No one going to press you about it.

SUSIE: I can't imagine anyone putting you on the spot: "I bet you've been masturbating with your comb and that's why you won't lend it to me!"

"MY FIANCÉ WON'T STAND FOR DIRTY TALK"

DEAR ARETHA & SUSIE,

I've been in a relationship for over three years, and for the past year we've been talking about getting married.

Since these conversations started, my boyfriend has begun to expect different things of me sexually. He gets upset if I use "dirty" words like *cock, pussy,* or *fuck.* He said, "The mother of my future children doesn't talk like that."

We're having less sex, and the sex we do have is more vanilla. I like vanilla sex, but I would like it more frequently. I'm afraid that he isn't seeing me as a sexual person anymore. If we do get married, I wonder if this will lead him to cheat.

One of the things that I liked about our relationship before, was that we had a great sexual connection—and he told me over and over how important sex is to him. So if he can't get it from me, will he look elsewhere? Help! *—Unhappy Angel in the House*

SUSIE: I wouldn't want him to be the father of my children, that's for sure.

ARETHA: You're worried about him cheating; I'm more worried about about how controlling he is. He's "Madonna-fying" you.

SUSIE: And you obviously don't want the prayer candle, you want your hot man back. I don't relish saying this, but what if he's already cheating on you? His libido didn't just disappear. Where did his sex drive go?

ARETHA: Anyone who says "The Mother of My Children Doesn't…"— Deal breaker.

"MY SWEET CHURCH-GOING HUSBAND WANTS ME TO ACT LIKE A PORN STAR IN BED"

DEAR ARETHA & SUSIE,

I'm in my second marriage. I met both my husbands within the framework of a tight-knit conservative religion. My current husband and myself consider ourselves religious people, although we came to this level of religion as adults.

Before I became more religious, I had been sexually active in college. My first marriage ended for many reasons; because he cheated on me numerous times and he was clinically addicted to porn. In this first marriage, I refused any type of sex beyond missionary style, because a) our religion forbids the placement of sperm anyplace besides the vagina and b) my husband treated me like crap and having sex was like someone going to the bathroom on me.

My second marriage is AWESOME. My husband *loves* me passionately: physically and emotionally. We have all kinds of sex: oral, vaginal, and anal, with occasional rimming and spanking. I do these things because I love my husband and I love pleasuring him- but there are aspects of our lovemaking I feel uneasy about.

My husband asks occasionally for me to shave my pubic hair. Or he'll ask me to spit on his dick when giving him oral. He gets off on lots of gratuitous moaning. He likes this "porn-aesthetic" and I just divorced my ex-husband because he was addicted to porn.

If I broached this issue with my husband he would immediately back off because he's a sensitive guy. I don't have anyone within my community to discuss it. What's the best way to handle this? I want to be desired for who I am rather than how much I can act like a porn star   **—Not a Porn Star Wannabe**

ARETHA: Okay, wow. This is messy. She says herself that if she talked to her husband about it, he would back off. So what's the problem?

SUSIE: I agree. Putting the hot buttons aside…if he listens to her and loves her, then anything is up for discussion. That's what intimacy is about. Wouldn't she want him to confide in her, if he was feeling this alienated?

ARETHA: She doesn't say that the sex is amazing with her husband—I don't hear her saying anything about enjoying herself.

SUSIE: Yeah, I noticed that, too. She performs all this wild sex because she loves him and wants to make him happy… but that's not the same thing as knowing your own happy place. It's an untenable situation.

ARETHA: She says she wants to be loved for who she is… so who is she? She needs to figure out what she wants in the bedroom. She doesn't want to feel like she's a porn star- what does she want to feel like?

SUSIE: I don't buy the "porn addiction" meme—but whatever the problem was with her last husband, she was neglected. Lied to. That's enough anguish right there.

ARETHA: Okay, NPSW, so now you're with a new guy who gives you lots of attention. You love being cherished by him. His desire for you is all you ever dreamed. But you're not getting the sex you want, and you don't like what you've been doing sexually for him. How did this not come up before you tied the knot?

SUSIE: I blame your tight-knit conservative religion.

ARETHA: You throw in a lot about your religion… but it doesn't seem like your current husband takes the "sperm-only-in-the-vagina" thing very seriously—and neither do you, since you're going along with it. You just have to talk to him. You have to. The longer you wait with these things, the worse it is. He won't like hearing that you've been turned off by what he likes. Too bad. He needs to hear it now, because he won't change all on his own.

SUSIE: I'm just speculating, but if you don't have orgasms with him, it's time to 'fess up. Cut the "performance" crap. Have you had an orgasm, with any partner? What was your sex life like before your turn in faith? What's your solo sex life like? Is it good? Would you take a chance to try something authentic with him? What WOULD make you moan, for real?

ARETHA: And if you can't bring yourself to break the ice, I'd suggest NOT looking for your next boyfriend in a conservative little religion group.

SUSIE: It's a proven recipe for marital sexual disaster. Just ask your local GOP fellowship. I think you know what I'm talking about, or you wouldn't be writing us.

"HOW CAN I GET MY GIRLFRIEND TO SHAVE HER PUBIC HAIR?"

DEAR ARETHA & SUSIE,

I'm a 19-year-old guy who's been with my girlfriend for four years. The sex is great—she's willing and more then able—but her lack of personal grooming is an issue. She *does* woman-scape, but very little. I love giving her oral sex but her pubic hair has got to go! What can I do to get her to clean up?　　　　　　　　　**—Hair Freeman**

ARETHA: If you have the nerve to ask your lover to shave, be prepared. It's on the level of "you need to lose weight."

There is no asking "nicely."

SUSIE: What does "woman-scape" mean?

ARETHA: Shaving!

SUSIE: How can their sex be "great" and he "loves" going down on her, but then he gets uptight about something as trivial as her hair? If he has an erection, how bad can it be?

It makes me wonder if he's planning to get out a camera.

ARETHA: The only way it's going to happen is if he says something—and she's not going to like it.

SUSIE: Well, what if he said, "Would you shave ME?" Make it into his kinky fantasy, and maybe she'll join in the dare. It wouldn't be a "self-esteem" issue.

ARETHA: No, she's smart, she'll see right through that. If my boyfriend said to me, "Let's shave!"—I'd say, "WHY?"

Susie and Aretha Bright

If he said,"It would turn me on,"—I'd say, "OH REALLY."

SUSIE: What's so ridiculous is that there's a lot more guys who get off on even the slightest glimpse of pubic hair...

ARETHA: Then how come we don't hear guys talking about the hotness of pubic hair, only tits and ass?

SUSIE: It's bravado... how many people say their real sexual preferences in public? Most guys aren't Adrian Colesberry.

ARETHA: To be honest, if I were her lover, I can imagine having my preferences about her pubic hair... but if she isn't the type of girl who's already waxing or shaving, then she's not that type—leave it alone.

If you stop going down on her all of sudden, that's trouble too. She'll know something's up.

SUSIE: I just noticed... you two have been going out for four years— why is it a problem NOW? You would think you'd be so close at this point that anything could come up; you could say anything.

ARETHA: If you made it through high school, the worst is over—you oughta be able to talk about pubic hair by now.

"THE WORD THAT DESCRIBES
ME IS SICK"

DEAR SUSIE AND ARETHA,

I experienced my first orgasm last year. No physical stimulation was involved—it was purely a mental exercise.

Since then, I've bought sex toys and used them with great success. I'm confident when it comes to my ability to please myself. The problem is the mental stimulation it takes to get me to come is the most depraved type. I'm not kidding. I'm worried that there's something wrong with me.

My fantasies don't involve death or mutilation, but that's about the only limit. I can't come, even with intense physical stimulation, unless I think about pain, humiliation, and obedience. I saw a list of fantasies that "cross the line" on some web site, and I think I hit at least two or three.

It's not just S&M. I find that fantasies of misogyny work just as well as ones of bondage, if not better—and I'm an unapologetic feminist. I know I shouldn't be ashamed to be sexual, but I think the word that describes me is "sick."

It doesn't help that I go to a women's college. I have about as much chance of finding a boyfriend as I do of winning the lottery. I don't know if I'll ever find it possible to achieve pleasure when I'm in a real relationship.

I'm not a virgin, but I've never come with another person. Is there a way to reconfigure your sex drive? Or am I asking for the equivalent of those deprogramming camps that certain awful parents send their gay kids to? Is there any help for a pervert like me?   —*One Sick Puppy*

ARETHA: Puppy, chill out. You are not sick.

SUSIE: Any credible sex-ed web site or book would take a more nuanced view of taboo fantasies than a "Don't Go There" list. Put down the *Cosmo*. You are hardly alone.

ARETHA: If you told me you got off thinking about sex with animals, being raped, incested, or anything else taboo—I still would not consider you sick. Fantasies about taboo things are great, because they are FANTASIES—nothing bad is happening in real life.

SUSIE: I'm sure there's been times in your life where you were made to do something you hated, or were humiliated by a bully or authority figure. No one finds it pleasant, let alone arousing. You have no control whatsoever. But when you fantasize an humiliating punishment, for example, or a depraved act—you control every aspect, every moment. You take yourself exactly to the erotic brink YOU want to go to... and then you get the catharsis, the orgasm. Lemonade is made out of your lemons. It's human nature.

ARETHA: What site did you go to that said certain fantasies "cross the line"—says WHO?

SUSIE: Yeah, you need to report them to the sex-ed police! The BEST research about why we fantasize about the things we *do* fantasize about, is in a book called *The Erotic Mind* by Jack Morin. It's worth a good ten years of therapy—and you'll be able to help a lot of other people feeling similarly tortured!

ARETHA: I have to ask, if she REALLY doesn't like these fantasies and wants to be thinking about something else—is there something else she could be doing?

SUSIE: It's not dog training. You can control behavior, but you cannot bend the unconscious to your will. Nobody likes to hear it, but that's the truth. When behavioral psychiatrists treat "repeat sex offenders"— people who cross the line of reality and consent, who violate other people's boundaries—they give them strict homework to masturbate to "appropriate" fantasy material and "aversion therapy" for the unwanted fantasies. The results have not been inspiring, much like the failures of the "Homo Rehab" camps. You can't suppress specific sex fantasies effectively. You can only diminish or eliminate one's entire libido by chemical or hormonal means. I'm sure that's not what Puppy has in mind!

ARETHA: Pup, I know you're at a women's college, but are you chained to your desk? Why do you think you can't have a boyfriend till graduation? Are all the other girls at your college waiting till graduation to have a bf, too?

SUSIE: Hitch a ride into town.

ARETHA: I don't know why you haven't come before with your other sexual partners, but I'm guessing they didn't know what turns you on.

SUSIE: I'm guessing you haven't had enough chances to try much of anything out—or some decent privacy!

ARETHA: Do you want to role-play your fantasies with a lover? Or even talk about them?

SUSIE: I predict you're going to find some really hot radical tender boyfriend who will be thrilled to find out you have the same "sick" fantasies that he does. Think up a funny "safe word" while you're sitting in your next semester of Abnormal Psychology. Don't waste another moment doubting yourself.

"I CAN'T SEPARATE SEX FROM MY EMOTIONS"

DEAR ARETHA & SUSIE,

I'm in a one-year-long exclusive relationship with a guy I like. We're friendly, funny, goofy, intimate, all that good stuff—and the sex is pretty good too.

We both want to sleep with other people occasionally, and don't really know what to do about it. He keeps suggesting an open relationship. We live together and I have a feeling that I would find it emotionally messy, even though his take is that it would only be occasional one-night stands.

I'm uneasy because there's part of me that's envious of his ability to separate sex from emotions (or so he says).

My abilities in compartmentalizing are a little limited, but I'm thinking it might be worth it to explore and find out. I don't think it's impossible. I feel "mentally" open but my stomach tells me otherwise, due to some lingering jealousy and an inherent and learned sense of loyalty.

Also, I live in a country that isn't exactly free-love-friendly so I can't expect acceptance from my peer group. Cheating is common here but I'm not interested in deception and jealousy. I don't have any positive role models when it comes to an open relationship.

Should I pursue this? He says he doesn't want to push the idea and will back off entirely if I say I'm not comfortable with it. He's loyal, honest, and patient, so the decision is up to me. Where should I begin? **—Wants to Open Up**

ARETHA: Well! This cracked me up because all I could think was, "My mom could tell you a lot more about this than I can!"—Lol.

SUSIE: Yeah, *har-de-har-har.*

ARETHA: Thinking about what happened with my Mom and Dad made me want to caution this girl that picking *who* you decide to open your relationship to, is super-duper important. Stay away from needy stalker people who want more than you can give them.

SUSIE: In my defense… in the 21 years I've been with your dad—all of which were non-monogamous—I can only think of two (and in retrospect, mercifully brief) times that we went through some real grief over other lovers. I don't blame it on being "open"—it's just the hard stages relationships go through at times, be they social, platonic, or battles with your own relatives.

You were our daughter, and part of the deal was you never knew about all the times everything worked out fine. We protected our family life: Children come first, privacy is a big deal, and discretion is definitely the better part of valor.

As to Miss Wanna-Be-Poly here, I'd say that the ideal time to find out about how you feel about open relationships is *definitely* before you have children.

ARETHA: But I don't think she's quite there yet—she's still deciding whether she wants to do it.

SUSIE: There are ways to get your feet wet. You could go to a play party together, and either watch, play, or both. Connect with other experienced lovers, or pros, for that matter. Avoid the ring-seeking singles and unhappily married. You could plan a "when-I'm-out-of-town" adventure, where what happens in Vegas stays in Vegas.

Talk about all the details, like where it happens, what happens the day after, what birth control or STD stuff you use.

There is no such thing as "disconnecting" your emotions, thank goodness. Would it please you to hear a little bit about his love life away from you, a lot, or nothing at all? If one of you is on a date, what does the other one do? Discuss how you feel about friends versus acquaintances, boys vs. girls, etc.

Each one of you reserves the right to change your mind. You already understand the most important thing: Open relationships are about Not Cheating. Not deceiving. Not patronizing your partner by keeping a secret.

ARETHA: I say, go for it. You've been together for a year, he's a loyal and honest guy, and you both want to sleep with other people; that's a great base. If you have the hots for some awesome guy and want to hook up with him—in an open relationship, that can happen! And it's NOT CHEATING. If you two try it for a month or whatever and you don't like it, then make sure he knows right away!

On the other hand... If your tummy is telling you that you're not up for it, then maybe you aren't ready. There is nothing wrong with that. Maybe just having the IDEA of sleeping with other people works for you better.

SUSIE: Good point. There are plenty of couples who get stoked on the fantasy of cheating, cuckolding, and "play" jealousy. You can go wild without bringing a single other live person into it.

Do you like to read your way into things? I do. Here's a reading list that'll get you thinking about the possibilities: *The Ethical Slut*, Tristan Taormino's *Opening Up*, and a short story I wrote for *Mommy's Little Girl*, called *"The Best She Ever Had."*

By the way.... I assume the UNfriendly-free-love locale you're describing is: The United States? Where is our utopia?

SCORNED BUT STILL HORNY

DEAR ARETHA AND SUSIE,

My long-distance boyfriend of two years broke up with me in June. We'd been having problems for a while, but I didn't think that he would end up dumping me.

In my post-breakup trauma, I've gone back to look at some emails we exchanged in the weeks before breaking up. At first, he insinuated that our relationship would "change" when I moved to LA from New York.

Then he started talking about "taking a break." One of the emails refers to a phone conversation where he said we could still have sex "as friends."

Now that I'm starting to accept he broke up with me, the ONLY thing I'm hoping for is the sex. I know it may seem silly, but the sex was amazing. I am aware of all "do-it-yourself" options, and frankly, I still just want him to give it to me.

Even though he said before that we could still have sex as "friends" (whatever that means), I'm afraid that when I confront him about it, he'll play dumb and reject me again.

How can you convince an ex that all you want is the sex and nothing more? Will men *ever* turn down sex that they know is reliably good?

I have planned a trip to see him for the first time in three months—and I plan on getting some. Please advise me on how to.

—*Scorned But Horny*

ARETHA: Being dumped, especially when you don't see it coming, is the worst.

SUSIE: Recapturing hot sex from a lost romance isn't reliable. You can't put it back in the bottle.

Susie and Aretha Bright

ARETHA: You remember the sex being amazing, but the sex will not be the same. After having been dumped only two-plus months ago, you put yourself at a lot of emotional risk—like being rejected (again) by him.

SUSIE: Even if he doesn't push you away... the dissonance between your old familiarity and the recent betrayal will leave your head spinning.

ARETHA: I think it would be far more healing for you to have wonderful sex—with someone else.

SUSIE: I second that motion. There ought to be a escort service for the recently-dumped.

Go ahead and have as many cathartic jill-off sessions as you want, thinking about him, coming, crying. Now that's reliable. Your dreams, your unconscious, have to work through it; there's no shortcut. Each little solitary orgasm and teardrop helps you find some peace.

ARETHA: I hate to crush your hope. But I want to discourage you from planning a trip to "get some"—I don't want you feeling bad.

SUSIE: Truth? I doubt you'll follow our advice. Both of us were once given the same counsel ourselves... and *ignored* it.

Your mother, your best friends, and all the sexperts will unanimously tell you to stay away. But it's like telling a child not to put a bean up their nose.

You want to pick the scab, you want to hold your finger in the flame, and this compulsion will remain attractive until one day you wake up and say: "I am too old for this."

Self-preservation will eventually kick in.

ARETHA: Part of me wants to give you wild advice about how to seduce him back into your bed, like, I dunno... Tell him you just want closure, then get him drunk and spike his cocktail with Viagra.

But NO! You need to pine, stay away, and GET OVER HIM. The

hurt feelings will feel better as time goes on, I promise.

SUSIE: Pine, stay away, masturbate, cry, and have some really smokin' sex with someone else. There is life after Mr. Wonderful!

"I'VE BEEN FAKING IT
ALL THIS TIME"

DEAR ARETHA & SUSIE,

I've been happily with a guy for two years. We have great, wonderful, passionate sex—but I never orgasm. Well, occasionally small ones. He doesn't know this. He thinks I have multiples and he's happy with the moaning and screaming. I'm happy with what I have. We have long sessions, they're very pleasurable, and I end up weak in the knees afterwards.

I use the metaphor that climaxing is like finally arriving at a cake shop down the street. Yeah, it's great to get there—and see a triple layer staring back at you. But if there's a carnival along the way to the cake shop, it ends up pale and unsatisfying by comparison.

I enjoy it so much more during the sessions when I DON'T climax and just hover in that nice feeling before an orgasm. Even when I'm going at it solo, climaxing is a hinderance.

I'm guilty for not telling him all this. I know it would make him feel bad, like he isn't doing a good job. He would feel like a lesser lover because he can't make me cum. I want to be able to tell him, because this is the only thing I've withheld from him or lied about. But I don't think he'll believe me if I tell him that orgasms suck and he makes me much happier without them. I don't want to undermine the relationship. **—In Love With Foreplay**

ARETHA: I swear. Again with the "We have great, wonderful, passionate sex!" right in the first sentence. Why is it that the people who write to us with problems always have the best sex?

SUSIE: Because they're romantic and hopeful. And so are we. The hopeless and cynical are not reading or writing.

ARETHA: Well, my first reaction was: She's fucked. Once you've had your first fake orgasm there's no going back. She's been fucking this guy for two YEARS! That's a lot of fake orgasms.

If she tells him all those moaning, screaming orgasms didn't really happen, their love-life is going to SUCK afterward. He WILL feel bad.

Ms. Foreplay, I'm not sure know why you feel guilty about this, after years of silence, but I say keep it to yourself. You want to stay with this guy and still have weak-in-the-knees sessions? Say nothing. It sounds like you are having a great time in bed and whatever your BF is doing is working for you.

SUSIE: Something about this doesn't add up.

I want to know more about orgasms you search for when you masturbate. Do you AVOID climaxing when you're by yourself? Have you had other lovers that brought you more intense pleasure?

Orgasm is simply a release of sexual energy. We all love being on "the edge;" it's the icing on everyone's cake-but you can only sustain it for so long. The volcano has to blow. The contractions bring you down, the blood flow subsides, and you enter the technical phase called "resolution." There is a relief that is sometimes sad, but always sweet.

Let me give you a visual: look at the illustrations - (page 50 is where I want you to start!—then go back and read everything)- of what orgasm does, anatomically, in *A New View of a Woman's Body*.

My speculation is that you are NOT at plateau; you are enjoying the early stages of excitement with your boyfriend- which are pleasurable. You've struggled, unhappily, to reach a higher level of intensity. You get thwarted as you enter the plateau phase and wish you had stayed in the shallow end. It's a nasty, cranky place.

You think you're going to be happy this way for the rest of your life? No. You've been rationalizing and trying to "make do."

I wish you would experience the deep end of pleasure, the whole orgasmic spectrum—if you haven't already—on your own. Then think about what it would take to share it with your lover.

ARETHA: You could start having sex with him and telling him afterward that you didn't cum but it still felt great. Tell him about the cake shop or whatever and make it sound positive and sexy—he may come around to the idea.

This would be an excellent time to try NEW things in bed- and I'm thinking of a few ways cake could be incorporated, too.

Don't get into "what if you told him everything?"—even though it would be "honest." It's a lot of hassle over the idea that sex is not good without an orgasm. I say skip it. Mom, you may disagree...

SUSIE: No, I agree with you... he won't buy it—and he'd be right. If he gets educated about female orgasm, he'll never buy it. It sounds like a two year grudge. He'll wonder, "Why now?"

Maybe that's the unspoken problem here. What's changing inside you? Are you having second thoughts about other things?

ARETHA: Ummm... and yeah! Your boyfriend sounds great. "Long sessions"? If he dumps you over the no-orgasm thing, give me his number!

SUSIE: That is so sisterly of you.

"HE GOES LIMP AT THE THOUGHT OF INTERCOURSE"

DEAR ARETHA & SUSIE,

My problem is so rare, that none of my trusted advisers have any idea what to do.

I recently started dating a younger guy—there's a seven year difference between us. We are getting along great: he's sweet, intelligent, gorgeous and we share a lot of interests. We're having great sex... sort of.

He's only been in a few relationships in his life. One lasted five years. But since he broke up with her—ages ago—he's been single and celibate. When our intimacy started, he told me he didn't like oral sex or intercourse.

I was stunned but tried to be understanding. We've been using our hands a lot—and after some pleading, he allowed me to perform oral sex with him, going very slowly over several weeks. Now he likes it and even requests it—but I still haven't been able to get him off that way.

He goes limp at even the THOUGHT of intercourse. I've asked him if he had a bad experience or if he finds vaginas gross. He swears he doesn't—it just doesn't do anything for him; he's always been that way. We've tried using foreplay to get him in the mood but when we try to actually do it, he loses his erection.

We've gotten close and I really want to share this with him. I don't want to "force" him into intercourse or have it all the time. But I want to at least try it once! If he can handle it or even likes it a little, it would be nice to have as an option. He says his body won't cooperate.

Other than this, our sex life is fine. We have sex all the time and it's great. If he never got over this, I'd be cool with it because he's really worth it. But I would be wistful for intercourse.

Possible related factors? He's uncut. He's not experienced. He's had confidence problems in the past. His last girlfriend was borderline emotionally abusive to him—but he's short on any details.

My strategy has been to be understanding and not obsess over it. I keep telling him: "We'll try it one day when you are really horny, have a raging hard-on, and it will work out—you'll get over whatever psychological stumbling block is there. Don't worry. I mean, we got over the oral sex thing, right?"

Any insight would be appreciated.   *—Patty Puzzled*

ARETHA: I hardly know where to start. My first reaction is: "HE'S GAY."

SUSIE: Ha! The last time I said that to *you*, Aretha, during a period of... uh... your romantic frustration—you said, "Mom, you don't know what you're talking about."

ARETHA: Well, you didn't! But I'm right about this.

SUSIE: How about putting it a more inclusive way; Patty's boyfriend doesn't conform to hetero-normative behavior. Which would be okay, if he was forthcoming and enthusiastic about his tastes—but he isn't.

There's one thing worse than him not fucking her, and that's him not talking straight with her. Is he even honest with himself?

ARETHA: Yeah, like what DOES he like? I cannot figure it out. It doesn't sound like he's got any other proximity issues, if the two of them are going at it with their hands. That being said—he can't get off from oral sex—and he can't stay hard enough to perform intercourse?

Patty sounds like a saint.

SUSIE: Saints don't make good sex-positive role models.

I have to say, I don't understand the hand action.

Puzzled, does he get you off with his hands? Does he go down on YOU? Does he like anal sex, in either direction? What does he do when he masturbates? How do you come? What are his fantasies?

ARETHA: Yeah, good questions. If your boyfriend can tell you what he doesn't like, he should be mature enough to tell you what he does like. If he was a virgin, it would be one thing—but this guy already had a five-year relationship with someone else.

SUSIE: He is a secret spun inside a secret. He wants you to play his beard but it's an intractable situation. Whether he has a history of abuse, (which we haven't even gotten into here) or is just too frightened to share his bent, you're not helping him—you're enabling a course in denial.

ARETHA: Enough about *him*! Puzzled, you say that even if you never have intercourse with him, you'd still hang on to him because such a swell guy—but you'd be wistful.

I'm thinking: *miserable.*

It's super-romantic right now. His inability to fuck might be a turn—on in some ways. I'm thinking... Marilyn Monroe and Tony Curtis in *Some Like It Hot.* But these feelings won't last long-term. Resentment and sexual frustration are around the corner.

SUSIE: I've known a few couples who didn't give a fig about intercourse. What they had in common was a great deal of sexual sophistication and a matching set of kinky appreciations. They wanted to be tied up, they wanted to 69 all day, they wanted to role-play and cross-dress. They weren't avoiding anything; they were going for their gusto. You don't meet many young people like that. It takes time and wisdom to come out of the closet.

Women are brought up to think that if it's "true love," they'll have baby-making sex. Lovers who throw that overboard work through a lot of baggage. They say bye-bye to the Harlequin Romances.

Not only do you have to have the political frame of reference, you need a sex drive that propels you outside the box. That doesn't sound like where you're coming from. You want your man inside you. You shouldn't be begging and hoping.

ARETHA: It sounds like she's tried everything obvious in the bedroom, and it's not working. I wonder if he has seen a doctor or a therapist?

SUSIE: I doubt he has; he's using Puzzled as a surrogate. It's not fair, to her or himself. Miss Puzz, you need your sexual self-interest addressed, and so does Hand Puppet. Listen to your "wistful" voice… it's trying to tell you something.

TOO FAT FOR SEX?— OR TOO CRAZY?

I am 20 years old and I'm a virgin. Usually it doesn't bother me, but lately I've had the feeling that something is wrong with me. The problem isn't that nobody will fuck me, or even that nobody I'm attracted to will fuck me.

I'm 5'4", 240 pounds, and it makes me feel completely neutered.

I can honestly say I've never felt sexy in my life! If someone tries to get close to me, I become so self-conscious that I withdraw. I don't know what to do.

The obvious answer is lose weight, and I'm working on it, but part of me knows that the weight is just the peak of my self-esteem iceberg. How can I get over this? Do I just need a ton of therapy?

—Bummer City

ARETHA: I think you are smart to point out that it's not your weight that's the base problem; it's a self-esteem issue.

SUSIE: There are fat women who are digging sex and falling in love. There are 36-24-36-type individuals who are alone in their room, depressed, so shy they don't know where to begin.

ARETHA: You gotta say, "I'm good enough, I'm smart enough, and gosh-darn it, people like me!"

SUSIE: I think seeing the entire *Stuart Smalley* movie is essential, at least once a year.

ARETHA: Look, fuck the weight calculations for now. Look around at what else is going on in your life... are you getting outside and getting enough exercise? Do you feel rested in the morning; do you have a fulfilling diet?

SUSIE: I'd encourage you to think of your "neutered" feelings as a health symptom. Are you depressed in other respects? Have you talked to any health-care pros about your medical history? How is your weight—or other issues, which you haven't mentioned—affecting your life? The sex stuff is one clue.

You have to go at this thing holistically... it's not your size versus your sexiness. Your "absence of feeling" is distressing. But you don't need a "ton" of therapy... you need a plan and small steps. And some help to do it. Your weight is just one part of it. These things are too hard to do alone. We're so far away... I want you to have people on your side, listening and helping you, who are closer than an email.

ARETHA: Do you masturbate? If you don't, I would recommend that you try it. The first step should be all about finding pleasure with yourself before you start tangling with other people and all their issues. When you're alone and you're feeling horny, there's no one else in the room to make you feel self-conscious, right? I say, get wild!

Throw away all your icky expectations about what you should be like, what you should be doing, and just try to enjoy being yourself.

I KNOW, easier said than done.

SUSIE: But what else is there? You're on the verge... you already know you can't go on like you've been.

ARETHA: The next time you're with someone and they try to "get close"—and you find yourself pulling away—try to notice what you're doing and PAUSE, just for a second!

Ask yourself, "Do I feel safe?"

"Do I want to withdraw or do I feel like I need to withdraw because that's what I always do?"

"Am I going to be okay if I just stay in the moment with this other person?"

And if you end up pulling away, that's fine. The point would be

that you knew what you were doing, and you made a conscious decision instead of just letting your self-esteem steer you around.

"ANTI-DEPRESSION DRUGS KILLED MY LIBIDO"

DEAR ARETHA & SUSIE,
A year and half ago I was put on Paxil to treat my crippling panic attacks and ever-worsening agoraphobia. It worked great! No more panic attacks...but also no more orgasms and a seriously decreased libido.

I read that those side effects usually went away within a couple months, but with me, they didn't. Earlier this year I went off the Paxil for a few reasons (like my orgasms and libido) and it was amazing. I was afraid I'd lost the ability to orgasm, but after I'd been medication-free for a few weeks, I was able to come hard, and multiple times. For a couple of months I masturbated every day, and enjoyed it so much. However, the panic attacks and anxiety came back. I went back on the Paxil.

I've been in a new relationship for the past two months. It's the best sex I've ever had, and I get a lot of pleasure out of it, but it is frustrating not to orgasm. I would love to be able to come with my new partner. Within the past month, I've even decreased my dose of my medication from 20mg to 10mg, hoping it would help—it hasn't.

The only way I can come is if he goes down on me and I need a lot of stimulation—clitoral and vaginal. Even then I don't always get there. I've had a few orgasms this way—it takes a long time, but I am always ecstatic when it does happen.

I suppose my question is, why do SSRIs have this side effect? What can I do to combat it while on the medication? I'm 22 years old; I don't want to be having sexual problems right now!

I cannot switch my medication or see my doctor. I am off of my parents' health insurance because I'm not a full time student this semester, so I'm restricted from my doctor and switching my medication. Ideally, I would like to see a therapist and deal with my panic disorder through therapy, but that's not a possibility right now

—Grace

ARETHA: You had to READ about the side effects of Paxil? They should have been the first words out of your doctor's mouth when you discussed an anti-depressant.

Paxil freaks me out. I had some friends in high school who were on Paxil until everyone found out that Paxil caused a significant number of children and young adults to have suicidal thoughts, and in some cases, suicide. You're under 25? You should read this.

Frankly, if you're only having problems with your libido, I think you are getting off light.

SUSIE: These are complicated drugs. And you're newly in love with your boyfriend... you have motive to be concerned about your relationship's future.

Grace, there's a reason you haven't easily found out the why's and wherefores of SSRI's. These drugs and their mental health effects were discovered almost by accident, and physiologists are still arguing about why they work—or why the results are so different for each patient. Everyone taking SSRI's today is a guinea pig.

I am not cavalier about your mental health issues—panic and anxiety can bring your life to a halt. The irony is, Paxil itself is something to be anxious about.

ARETHA: The best thing you can do is see a doctor and describe these issues. And get your prescription changed. Period. I would recommend seeing a different doctor next time! I understand you don't have any health insurance, so unless you can pay for a doctor's visit out-of-pocket—you are indeed in a fix.

SUSIE: You're dependent on your parents for health care. They probably care for you dearly, and you may have other devoted family, as well. These people give a damn about your health. Your panic attacks are of great concern to them—they would care if the treatment you're receiving is making you ill.

Face it, if you broke your leg, your family wouldn't say, "Too bad, you're only a part-time student, you can just stay home and make your own cast."

I know you're thinking, "I can't tell my parents, 'it's an emergency, my sex life is bumming out on Paxil.'" I understand that sexual dysfunction is considered a trivial pursuit by some, not essential to your physical or mental health. Even you act like, "Hey, I can get by."

I would encourage you to think of your entire brain stem and cerebral cortex with more care. Your difficulty with orgasms is symptomatic of enormous changes. Your testosterone may be down, your prolactin may be up, your Paxil is a vaso-constrictor that affects your blood stream as well as your synapses. The action of SSRI's suppresses the engorgement of erectile tissue.

If you tell your family, "I'm getting some relief with Paxil, but there's some weird side effects that are sickening me and I've been reading things too... I want to see a doctor ASAP"—would they refuse you?

If they do refuse (!!!) you need to investigate your school's health clinic. Find out what kind of nutrition, aerobics, meditation, and life-coping skills classes are being offered on your campus at little or no cost to students. Each one of these topics is a serious book on response to anxiety and panic attacks. Your school's medical staff deals with thousands of students who are battling to stay in school because of mental health problems; they discuss these issues all the time. What about low-cost therapy?

ARETHA: I'm familiar with your story about taking "drug holidays" where you STOP taking their drug for a couple of days to get their libido back. Sounds like you already took a long vacation, and you saw what happened. Ideally, all these different approaches should be consulted with a doctor before you do anything, of course!

SUSIE: It can be problematic to wean off Paxil. You were lucky.

ARETHA: I notice you say you're having the best sex you've ever had.

SUSIE: Long luxurious cunnilingus... yeah, other people are drooling at your sexual dilemma.

ARETHA: So, maybe things aren't too bad in the present.

SUSIE:—At least the short term sex effects. I'm more concerned about the big picture. If I was your mommy, I'd have you in a qualified psychologist's office faster than you can say "dopaminergic neurotransmission."

ARETHA: Until next semester!

THE SLUT FACTOR

DEAR SUSIE AND ARETHA,

At what point is promiscuity self-destructive? At what point is it empowering?

—*Carrie*

ARETHA: It depends on the people you're sleeping with! No jealous jerks, psychos, disrespectful people. Keep a standard. Know what you're attracted to, and don't fuck just anybody.

SUSIE: Well, that would be easy if you could tell all of that ahead of time. What about the other side, how do you know if it's empowering?

ARETHA: Having as much sex as you want is empowering when you're having fun, you're eating, sleeping, working, getting on with your life.

SUSIE: I love that you always put *sleeping* on your "Top 5" list.

I have a problem with that word, "promiscuity." It implies sluttyness, which is used to shame women, not men.

It's not what the town prude thinks about you that's the issue, it's whether you're having satisfying reciprocal sex with people who respect sex itself.

"IF I DON'T FEEL PRETTY
I CAN'T `GET AROUSED"

DEAR ARETHA & SUSIE,

Here's the thing: I've realized I haven't figured out sex yet.

I've never had an orgasm. All I want to do is make my boyfriend happy, put him in blissy-eyed nirvana, and impress him with my tight body. I like it but it's vanity—I want to be a good lay for him. Sex from the female perspective bores me. I can't imagine physical pleasure that would be appealing for its own sake.

This has its downside. I secretly wish my boyfriend to come as soon as possible so we can stop. If I don't feel pretty, I can't get aroused. I can't masturbate—after all, there's nobody to impress if I'm alone.

When I was growing up, I was a "brain" and boys didn't notice me. Now men do notice me—and I like it—but I'm ashamed how badly I've come to need their attention.

I'm sure some of this will go away over time. I'm 21 and I've only slept with one person. But I could use a little help. My boyfriend has actually asked me to enjoy his body more. He wants me to ask him to do things for me, but I just can't. I want to be wanted—terribly, fearfully—and I have no goddamn idea what I want myself.

M'aidez! I'm so tired of being sexually dependent.   **—Unblissed**

ARETHA: It's time to brainwash yourself the other way around.

Here's the thing: Your boyfriend wants you to get off. Period! Men think it's AROUSING when women enjoy themselves in bed. It sounds like he's already been dropping you hints.

SUSIE: They're more than hints. Your BF is desperate. Did he write this letter for you?

Most lovers find it so difficult to ask for anything in bed, that if it rises to the level of a kind request, you can be sure he's been obsessing about it for hours, wondering how to break the ice.

ARETHA: Have you told your boyfriend your feelings or is it a secret?
SUSIE: He'd find it enlightening to hear what you told us. Could you bring yourself to confide in him? Not in bed, but with your clothes on and all your wits about you.

This isn't going to disappear. Even your vanity is boring you. You're faced with deciding if this fellow is a treasure to cherish—or if you're moving onto the next "impressionable" young thing. Without your own pleasure, the superficial ego strokes are going to seem more and more paltry.

ARETHA: You say that you can't find any physical pleasure that would be appealing, that's just for you.

What about... if your boyfriend gave you a massage? Or made you something delicious to eat?

Both of those things are also physical sensations that make you feel good, just like sex. Think of that the next time you're in bed with him. I know it can be hard to receive "the goods" when you're used to being the giver—so start small.

The next time you two are in bed, don't think, "And now... I am going to FORCE myself to HAVE AN ORGASM." Instead, ask your BF to give you a nice back rub or something before the sex even starts and you go into your "mode."

Let yourself be spoiled, whether it's sexually, physically, or emotionally. In general, boyfriends LIKE to take care of their girlfriends and make them feel good, sexy, secure.

SUSIE: You've got one of those good ones in your bed right now.

I reviewed a book recently about a young woman's search for orgasm. Her disdain and cheeky humor about "not getting it" was all too familiar.

I wrote, "What does this lack of female orgasm mean? Is it like missing the Grand Tour of Europe—or the crosstown bus? Is it overrated?

The young author got one lucid answer from an expert she queried, who's also a colleague of mine—Dr. Rae Larson.

"'People overvalue orgasm,' Larson told her. "They go looking for an orgasm instead of pleasure. Look for pleasure first; that will lead you to where you want to go.'"

I'm not going to twist your arm and tell you about masturbation, the clitoral body, and the wonders of sexual self knowledge. You are obviously a well-read cookie.

Instead, find out what gives you a thrill. There is nothing boring about that. I don't care if it's pole-dancing, swimming in open water, bad porn, or jumping out of an airplane. You find out what makes your heart race, what makes you euphoric, what makes you involuntarily wet—and the orgasm will simply show up, a nervous system response to a well-lubricated limbic system.

"I'M A GIRL WHO COMES
TOO FAST"

DEAR ARETHA & SUSIE,

I have a frustrating sexual problem that masquerades as a blessing. I enjoy sex with my boyfriend of three years, and am able to orgasm every time. The problem is that I usually come in the first few minutes.

After this first orgasm, I just feel "done." It doesn't hurt to continue, but I lose interest in sex and my body seems to shut down to further stimulation. I've tried delaying my orgasm, but after penetration, there's only so long I can control myself without going down the path to orgasm.

While I can be perfectly happy with two-minute sex, my guy has stamina and wants to continue. He understands when I ask to stop—and he'll get off another way—but this mismatch in our timing makes it hard to stay connected during sex.

I'd also like to experience longer-lasting sex myself without a premature orgasm getting in the way. It's common to hear of men dealing with this problem, but as a woman, I don't know why I can't last during sex—or how come I can't keep going after my first orgasm.

What's the deal?

—**One Minute Woman**

ARETHA: Huh. Interesting.

I have random ideas of what could help… and a lot of questions!

After you come, are you "done" for an hour, or are you "done" for the day? Do you notice that you come quicker or slower depending on how often you and your boyfriend have sex? Do you ever masturbate and come before you have partner sex?

Have you tried different positions? Maybe something different that you normally don't do would help you last longer. Have you tried putting a pack of ice on your vagina? (Just kidding).

SUSIE: The icepack would definitely do it! I love this question. Men and women are so similar—and we're usually so focused on minute differences, we miss the big picture.

Women who are familiar with their lover and know what they like, often find that coming fast is easy. Too easy. You're confronted with the fact that you, Miss Considerate, feel like pushing the dude off of you, whampbam-thank-you-m'am. We can all be selfish piggies.

Like any guy facing this question, you have to ask yourself, "Do I give a darn?"

There is some self-interest involved... as Aretha said, you can tease out the foreplay, a little variety, and drive yourself delight-fully crazy. Make yourself beg for it before you give in... this can lead to some fun scenarios. That's what most women do in this situation. Doing algebra or baseball stats in your head is a little more perverse.

Or perhaps you'd like to give yourself wiggle room on the other end. You might not feel like doing ANYTHING in the first five minutes after coming, but try doubling or tripling that. When you come again, it will probably be slower but it might be more intense.

You've been with this guy for three years. You've probably laughed about being a "premie," or talked about it seriously at times. Furthermore, he must SEE what he does that drives you over the edge. Maybe he likes it that way, if he's so quick to oblige.

I would ask him, knowing each other as you do, what have been the best times for him, when it "clicked," timing-wise. Maybe you'll be surprised to compare answers.

No matter what you come up with, don't forget to reserve the special occasions for you to fly off the handle and start snoring in post-orgasmic slumber. How could anyone deny you that, every once in a while? I stand with you, in premature sisterhood.

AFTERWORD FROM THE MOTHER

The first time I tried to publish responsible sex advice, I was sixteen. The principal at my high school brought me into his office and said, "If you ever pull a stunt like this again, you'll be thrown out of school for good."

Guess which way I went?

It's funny to think about my first attempt at sisterly bedroom advice. The dilimma I picked is one of the most common female sexual complaints: "What do you do when sex hurts?"—when putting *anything* in your vagina feels dry, painful, and horrid?

I may have been a tenth-grader with almost-zero personal sex experience, but I did know the answer: *lack of lubrication*. I was a feminist bookworm—if just newly sexually active—and I knew all about it.

The main way a woman gets lubricated is by being aroused, and without it, penetration is torture. I decided to write a little essay on this pressing subject for the high school paper.

I did all the science parts first—how the vagina needs lubrication, and that if you're not generating it on your own, you need a little help—from vegetable oil or water-soluble lube. Back in the 1970s, that was K-Y jelly.

But!—the real sin, according to my Principal, was that I had added some homespun wisdom to my story. I wrote that if you couldn't get the money for lube, or were too shy to grab olive oil out of the kitchen—you could, at the very least, take some saliva from your mouth with your fingertips, and reach down there and make things moist.

"Saliva!" I remember him shouting, like I had just screamed SLOPPY CUNT from the rooftops. "You can't say that word!"

Oh yes I can.

Back in those days, most of the sex ed I did was as part of the women's lib consciousness-raising group" we held during recess on the Girl's Athletic Field. (Which we renamed, of course, the "Women's Athletic Field").

We were hell-raisers, that's for sure. We demanded birth control seminars on campus, self-defense and rape awareness workshops. We talked about sex all the time and encouraged each other to be adventurous. We turned a janitor's closet into an abortion and birth control referral center. *Our Bodies Ourselves* was our bible. I had memorized that book before I'd kissed nothing more than my pillow.

It would be another ten years before I became a sex education professional, counseling customers at the first feminist vibrator store, in San Francisco. By then, I knew that while a good below-the-waist anatomy lesson was essential, there were a lot of issues that were entirely about desire, the erotic life of the mind. That's where things get a little more tricky and a lot less literal.

To touch back on the "getting aroused" aspect of lubrication—if you're not turned on, or if you don't feel free to express yourself, it doesn't matter how much lube you pour on your clit.

I remember my first tormented customers at the vibrator shop. A woman would say to me, "I feel like a failure, I can't come, something is wrong with me."—Like she was all alone!

I'd take her hand. "You know, women everywhere feel this way. I'll tell you something, I've never met a man who said he couldn't find his penis and never had an orgasm.—Why do you think *that* is?"

That would make her laugh, and then think about how maybe the Double Standard had screwed up her sex life, not her natural rhythm.

Little girls get told all the time that "down there" is bad. Most girls don't even learn the word for their primary sex organ, *clitoris*, until they're past puberty. Can you imagine a little boy not knowing the name for his penis, and never having "touched it" in his whole life?

Young women too often are raised to be scared of sex, ashamed of desire—and warned that it will be our ruin. We act in America like we're so "advanced," but when you think about all the slut-shaming, Purity Balls, and moral panics over "virginity," it's obvious we're not that far along.

When Aretha and I started writing for *Jezebel*, I'd been a "sexpert" for everyone from *Marie Claire* to *On Our Backs* to *Playboy*. But this bloggers' audience of teenagers and 20-somethings at *Jez* was the most poignant assignment of all, like going back in a time machine.

The same things I had worried about when I was young—that it was hard to come, that I could never "do it "in front of my lover, that I was undesirable, clumsy, that my fantasies were weird—it was still the same! In fact it was worse, because unfortunately high schools and college campuses are not filled with women's libbers anymore. I was never slut-shamed or baited in high school by other girls; virginity was not on a pedestal.

Writing with Aretha was hilarious, enlightening. I'm not the kind of mom who pries into her daughter's' sex life—in fact, the problem of "nosy parents" is one of my pet peeves.

So the way I found out what Aretha thought about sex, truly, was listening to her reactions to the letters we got.

She had a take on things I had grown callous to—a joie de vivre that races the pulse of young adulthood. I was such a crusty by comparison—cynical with all my facts and figures, easily exasperated. She would be patient and creative, while I was having my perimenopausal "WHY BOTHER!" tantrums.

But when I was eighteen, I was that eager, too. She *made* me remember! Our arguments led to such better "sex ed" than if we had been seconding each other on every topic.

There were two issues I was unaccustomed to, a sign of the times, I believe. Some would just called it a good old-fashioned anti-feminist, sex-negative backlash.

One was that a significant part of our audience had previous or current experience with SSRI's, antidepressant drugs, which had had a deleterious effect on the sex lives. They wrote us, worried.

Aretha and I both took mental health issues very much to heart, but we knew the pitfalls and history of how women are medicated—for "hysteria," for depression, for everything, often with no more than a five-minute intake (as one of our letter-writers described).

When we detailed the hard questions about SSRI's some of our audience and colleagues went ballistic. I began to wonder if Big Pharma was planting moles, it got so bad. I was told, by one commenter (who reminded me of my old high school principal), that I had No Right to Comment on sexual health and medicine, because I wasn't a doctor.

"No, I'm a journalist and a whistleblower and an activist, and this is what I've been doing since high school." Any credible sex educator would do the same.

Another mystery: a few of our column critics mounted a campaign to say that Susie and Aretha Bright were *forcing* women to have orgasms "whether they wanted them or not"—that we were not giving women "a choice."

These women explained that they were amoebas (non-sexual) or preferred to have sex *without* orgasm, and that we were oppressing them with our interest in women's consummate pleasure. If they wanted to "lie there and think of England," they would not be denied!

Apparently the pressures of their family, church, and peers were a mere piffle compared to a single Bright column on the how to lend a gal a hand.

One advantage of age is that I don't take this argument at face value anymore. I see it more as the scaly green side of women divided against each other, shaming each other, letting the "little chicks fight among themselves"—over far too little and too late. If you think that I, David-like with my Magic Wand, am going to take down the Goliath of Patriarchy with a single buzz—well, I wish. I do give it my best shot.

The fact is, the finest thing I've ever done, sex advice-wise, is also the best counsel I've ever received.

It goes like this:

"I'm your friend and I care about you. Your sexual life is at your center—no one can ever take it away or turn it into a lie. It's always there, waiting for you. And I will be there for you, too, no matter what." If that doesn't pass the wet test, I don't know what does.

SUSIE BRIGHT
2012

SOME OF OUR FAVORITE
SEX EDUCATION AND ADVICE

A Kid's First Book About Sex, by Joani Blank

I Am My Lover, edited by Joani Blank

Our Bodies Ourselves, by The Boston Women's Health
Book Collective

Lesbian Health Matters, by Mary O'Donnell

A New View of a Woman's Body: A Fully Illustrated Guide,
by Suzann Gage et al.

The Clitoral Truth: The Secret World at Your Fingertips,
by Rebecca Chalker

The Ultimate Guide to Sex and Disability, edited by Miriam Kaufman, Cory Silverberg

Full Exposure, by Susie Bright

Love & Lust: A Guided Sex Journal, edited by Susie Bright

The Erotic Mind, by Jack Morin

S.E.X., by Heather Corinna

How to Make Love to Adrian Colesberry, by Adrian Colesberry

Ill-Equipped for a Life of Sex, by Jennifer Lehr

Opening Up: A Guide to Creating and Sustaining Open Relationships, by Tristan Taormino

Deal With It, by Rebecca Odes, Heather McDonald, Esther Drill

The Ultimate Guide to Cunnilingus by Violet Blue

The Survivor's Guide to Sex, Staci Haines

The Ultimate Guide to Anal Sex for Women, by Tristan Taormino

Ill-Equipped for a Life of Sex, by Jennifer Lehr

Good Vibrations Sex Book by Cathy Winks and Anne Semans

VIDEOS

Fire on the Mountain: Male Genital Massage, directed by Joseph Kramer

Healing Sex, directed by Staci Haines, author of *A Survivor's Guide to Sex*

Self-Loving: A Woman's Sexuality Seminar, directed by Betty Dodson

WEB SITES

San Francisco Sex Information: http://sfsi.org/

Scarleteen: http://Scarleteen.com

Go Ask Alice! : http://www.goaskalice.columbia.edu/

Planned Parenthood: http://www.plannedparenthood.org/info-for-teens/

Coalition for Positive Sexuality: http://www.positive.org/Home/index.html

Dan Savage, Savage Love: http://www.thestranger.com/seattle/SavageLove?oid=10480174

OTHER TITLES BY SUSIE BRIGHT

The Erotic Screen, Volume 1: The Golden Hardcore and the Shimmering Dyke-Core

Big Sex Little Death: A Memoir

Love and Lust: A Sex Journal

Bitten, Editor

X: The Erotic Treasury, Editor

The Best American Erotica, 1993-2008, Series Editor

Inspired By Andrea Dworkin: Essays on Lust, Aggression, Porn, & The Female Gaze That I Might Not Have Written If Not for Her

Mommy's Little Girl: On Sex, Motherhood, Porn, & Cherry Pie

Three Kinds of Asking For It, Editor

Three The Hard Way, Editor

How To Write a Dirty Story

Full Exposure

The Sexual State of the Union

Nothing But the Girl: The Blatant Lesbian Image, Co-edited and written with Jill Posener

Sexwise
Sexual Reality
Herotica, Herotica 2, Herotica 3

Susie Sexpert's Lesbian Sex World

Susie Bright's Journal: http://susiebright.com

www.ingramcontent.com/pod-product-compliance
Lightning Source LLC
Chambersburg PA
CBHW020343290526
45785CB00005B/2152